The Complete Keto Diet Vegetarian Recipes

Low Carb and Fast Recipes to Burn Fast and Boost your Metabolism

Otis Fisher

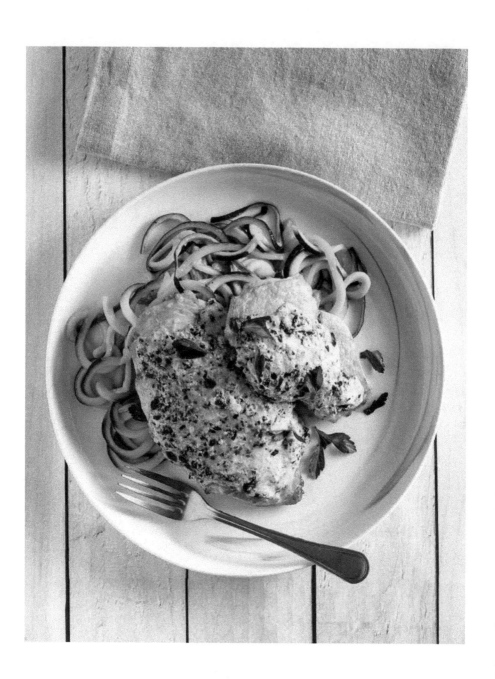

advice. The content within this book has been derived from various sources. Please consult a licensed professional before attempting any techniques outlined in this book.

By reading this document, the reader agrees that under no circumstances is the author responsible for any losses, direct or indirect, which are incurred as a result of the use of information contained within this document, including, but not limited to, — errors, omissions, or inaccuracies.

Table of contents

Broccoli and Almond Flour Chaffles

Preparation time: 6 minutes

Cooking Time: 8 Minutes

Servings: 2

Ingredients:

- 1 organic egg, beaten
- 1/2 cup Cheddar cheese, shredded
- 1/4 cup fresh broccoli, chopped
- 1 tablespoon almond flour
- 1/4 teaspoon garlic powder

Directions:

1. Preheat a mini Chaffle iron and then grease it.
2. In a bowl, place all ingredients and mix until well merged.
3. Set half of the mixture into preheated Chaffle iron and Cooking for about 4 minutes or until golden brown.
4. Repeat with the remaining mixture.
5. Serve warm.

Nutrition:

Calories 221

Protein 17 g

Carbs 31 g

Fat 8 g

Cheddar Jalapeño Chaffle

Preparation time: 6 minutes

Cooking Time: 5 Minutes

Servings: 2

Ingredients:

- 2 large eggs
- 1/2 cup shredded mozzarella
- 1/4 cup almond flour
- 1/2 tsp. baking powder
- 1/4 cup shredded cheddar cheese
- 2 Tbsp. diced jalapeños jarred or canned

For the toppings:

- 1/2 Cooked bacon, chopped
- 2 Tbsp. cream cheese
- 1/4 jalapeño slices

Directions:

1. Turn on Chaffle maker to heat and oil it with Cooking spray.
2. Mix mozzarella, eggs, baking powder, almond flour, and garlic powder in a bowl.
3. Sprinkle 2 Tbsp. cheddar cheese in a thin layer on Chaffle maker, and 1/2 jalapeño.

4. Ladle half of the egg mixture on top of the cheese and jalapeños.
5. Cooking for minutes, or until done.
6. Repeat for the second chaffle.
7. Top with cream cheese, bacon, and jalapeño slices.

Nutrition:

Calories 221

Protein 13 g

Carbs 1 g

Fat 34 g

Sodium 80 mg

Rosemary in Chaffles

Preparation time: 6 minutes

Cooking Time: 8 Minutes

Servings: 2

Ingredients:

- 1 organic egg, beaten
- 1/2 cup Cheddar cheese, shredded
- 1 tablespoon almond flour
- 1 tablespoon fresh rosemary, chopped
- salt and ground black pepper

Directions:

1. Preheat a mini Chaffle iron and then grease it.
2. For chaffles: In a medium bowl, place all ingredients and with a fork, mix until well merged.
3. Set half of the mixture into preheated Chaffle iron and Cooking for about 4 minutes or until golden brown.
4. Repeat with the remaining mixture.
5. Serve warm.

Nutrition:

Calories 221

Protein 12 g

Carbs 29 g,

Fat 8 g

Sodium 398 mg

Zucchini Chaffles with Peanut Butter

Preparation time: 5 minutes

Cooking Time: 5 Minutes

Servings: 2

Ingredients:

- 1 cup zucchini grated
- 1 egg beaten
- 1/2 cup shredded parmesan cheese
- 1/4 cup shredded mozzarella cheese
- 1 tsp. dried basil
- 1/2 tsp. salt
- 1/2 tsp. black pepper
- 2 tbsps. peanut butter for topping

Directions:

1. Sprinkle salt over zucchini and let it sit for minutes Utes.
2. Squeeze out water from zucchini.
3. Beat egg with zucchini, basil. salt mozzarella cheese, and pepper.
4. Sprinkle 1/2 of the parmesan cheese over preheated Chaffle maker and pour zucchini batter over it.
5. Sprinkle the remaining cheese over it.
6. Close the lid.

7. Cooking zucchini chaffles for about 4-8 minutes Utes.

8. Remove chaffles from the maker and repeat with the remaining batter.

9. Serve with peanut butter on top and enjoy!

Nutrition:

Calories 124

Protein 15 g

Carbs 0 g

Fat 7 g,

Zucchini in Chaffles

Preparation time: 10 minutes

Cooking Time: 18 Minutes

Servings: 2

Ingredients:

- 2 large zucchinis, grated and squeezed
- 2 large organic eggs
- 2/3 cup Cheddar cheese, shredded
- 2 tablespoons coconut flour
- 1/2 teaspoon garlic powder
- 1/2 teaspoon red pepper flakes, crushed
- Salt, to taste

Directions:

1. Preheat a Chaffle iron and then grease it.
2. In a medium bowl, set all ingredients and, mix until well combined.
3. Place 1/4 of the mixture into preheated Chaffle iron and Cooking for about 4-41/2 minutes or until golden brown.
4. Repeat with the remaining mixture.
5. Serve warm.

Nutrition:

Calories 311

Protein 16 g

Carbs 17 g

Fat 15 g

Garlic and Onion Powder Chaffles

Preparation time: 5 minutes

Cooking Time: 5 Minutes

Servings: 2

Ingredients:

- 1 organic egg, beaten
- 1/4 cup Cheddar cheese, shredded
- 2 tablespoons almond flour
- 1/2 teaspoon organic baking powder
- 1/4 teaspoon garlic powder
- 1/4 teaspoon onion powder
- Pinch of salt

Directions:

1. Preheat a Chaffle iron and then grease it.
2. In a bowl, set all the ingredients and beat until well combined.
3. Place the mixture into preheated Chaffle iron and Cooking for about 5 minutes or until golden brown.
4. Serve warm.

Nutrition:

Calories 249,

Protein 12 g

Carbs 30 g

Fat 10 g

Savory Bagel Seasoning Chaffles

Preparation time: 10 minutes

Cooking Time: 5 Minutes

Servings: 4

Ingredients:

- 2 tbsps. everything bagel seasoning
- 2 eggs
- 1 cup mozzarella cheese
- 1/2 cup grated parmesan

Directions:

1. Preheat the square Chaffle maker and grease with Cooking spray.
2. Mix together eggs, mozzarella cheese and grated cheese in a bowl.
3. Set half of the batter in the Chaffle maker.
4. Sprinkle 1 tbsp. of the everything bagel seasoning over batter.
5. Close the lid.
6. Cooking chaffles for about 3-4 minutes Utes.
7. Repeat with the remaining batter.
8. Serve hot and enjoy!

Nutrition:

Calories 64

Fat 3.1

Fiber 3

Carbs 7.1

Protein 2.8

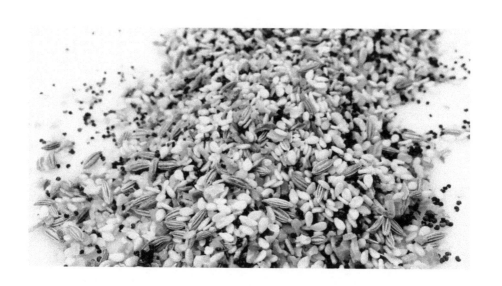

Dried Herbs Chaffle

Preparation time: 6 minutes

Cooking Time: 8 Minutes

Servings: 2

Ingredients:

- 1 organic egg, beaten
- 1/2 cup Cheddar cheese, shredded
- 1 tablespoon almond flour
- Pinch of dried thyme, crushed
- Pinch of dried rosemary, crushed

Directions:

1. Preheat a mini Chaffle iron and then grease it.
2. In a bowl, place all the ingredients and beat until well merged.
3. Set half of the mixture into preheated Chaffle iron and Cooking for about 4 minutes or until golden brown.
4. Repeat with the remaining mixture.
5. Serve warm.

Nutrition:

Calories 80

Fat 2.5

Fiber 3.9

Carbs 10.9

Protein 4

Zucchini and Basil Chaffles

Preparation time: 6 minutes

Cooking Time: 10 Minutes

Servings: 2

Ingredients:

- 1 organic egg, beaten
- 1/4 cup Mozzarella cheese, shredded
- 2 tablespoons Parmesan cheese, grated
- 1/2 of small zucchini, grated and squeezed
- 1/4 teaspoon dried basil, crushed
- Freshly ground black pepper, as required

Directions:

1. Preheat a mini Chaffle iron and then grease it.
2. In a medium bowl, set all ingredients and mix until well combined.
3. Set half of the mixture into preheated Chaffle iron and Cooking for about 4-5 minutes or until golden brown.
4. Repeat with the remaining mixture.
5. Serve warm.

Nutrition:

Calories 43

Fat 3.4

Fiber 1.7

Carbs 3.4

Protein 1.3

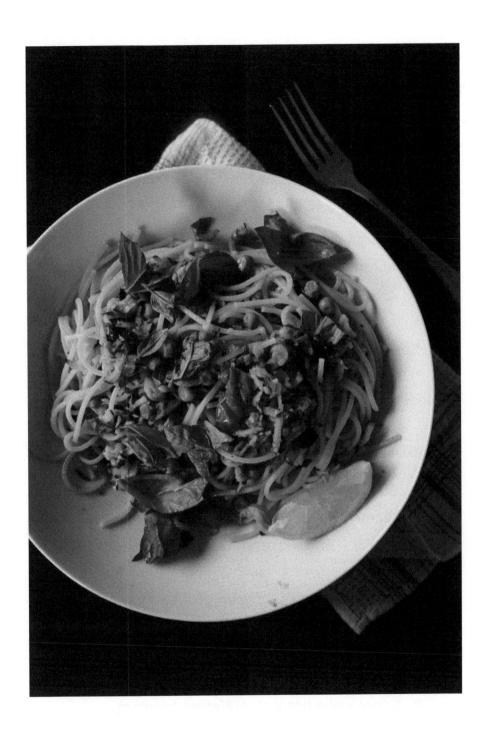

Hash Brown Chaffle

Preparation time: 6 minutes

Cooking Time: 10 Minutes

Servings: 2

Ingredients:

- 1 large jicama root, peeled and shredded
- 1/2 medium onion, minced
- 2 garlic cloves, pressed
- 1 cup cheddar shredded cheese
- 2 eggs
- Salt and pepper, to taste

Directions:

1. Place jicama in a colander, sprinkle with 2 tsp. salt, and let drain.
2. Squeeze out all excess liquid.
3. Microwave jicama for 5-8 minutes.
4. Mix 3/4 of cheese and all other ingredients in a bowl.
5. Sprinkle 1-2 tsp. cheese on Chaffle maker, add 3 Tbsp. mixture, and top with 1-2 tsp. cheese.
6. Cooking for 5-minutes, or until done.
7. Remove and repeat for remaining batter.
8. Serve while hot with preferred toppings.

Nutrition:

Calories 81

Fat 4.2

Fiber 6.5

Carbs 11.1

Protein 1.9

Cheese Garlic Chaffle

Preparation time: 10 minutes

Cooking Time: 8 Minutes

Servings: 2

Ingredients:

Chaffle

- 1 egg
- 1 teaspoon cream cheese
- 1/2 cup mozzarella cheese, shredded
- 1/2 teaspoon garlic powder
- 1 teaspoon Italian seasoning

Topping

- 1 tablespoon butter
- 1/2 teaspoon garlic powder
- 1/2 teaspoon Italian seasoning
- 2 tablespoon mozzarella cheese, shredded

Directions:

1. Plug in your Chaffle maker to preheat.
2. Preheat your oven to 350 degrees F.
3. In a bowl, combine all the chaffle ingredients.
4. Cooking in the Chaffle maker for minutes per chaffle.
5. Transfer to a baking pan.

6. Spread butter on top of each chaffle.

7. Sprinkle garlic powder and Italian seasoning on top.

8. Top with mozzarella cheese.

9. Bake until the cheese has melted.

Nutrition:

Calories 526

Fat 53.2

Fiber 7.8

Carbs 11.7

Protein 8.2

Cinnamon Cream Cheese Chaffle

Preparation time: 10 minutes

Cooking Time: 15 Minutes

Servings: 2

Ingredients:

- 2 eggs, lightly beaten
- 1 tsp. collagen
- 1/4 tsp. baking powder, gluten-free
- 1 tsp. monk fruit sweetener
- 1/2 tsp. cinnamon
- 1/4 cup cream cheese, softened
- Pinch of salt

Directions:

1. Preheat your Chaffle maker.
2. Attach all ingredients into the bowl and beat using hand mixer until well combined.
3. Spray Chaffle maker with Cooking spray.
4. Pour 1/2 batter in the hot Chaffle maker and Cooking for 3-minutes or until golden brown. Repeat with the remaining batter.
5. Serve and enjoy.

Nutrition:

Calories 60

Fat 30.7

Fiber 2.5

Carbs 6.4

Protein 2

Tomato Sandwich Chaffles

Preparation time: 10 minutes

Cooking Time: 6 Minutes

Servings: 2

Ingredients:

Chaffles

- 1 large organic egg, beaten
- 1/2 cup Colby jack cheese, shredded finely
- 1/8 teaspoon organic vanilla extract

Filling

- 1 small tomato, sliced
- 2 teaspoons fresh basil leaves

Directions:

1. Preheat a mini Chaffle iron and then grease it.
2. For chaffles: in a small bowl, place all the ingredients and stir to combine.
3. Set half of the mixture into preheated Chaffle iron and cooking for about minutes.
4. Repeat with the remaining mixture.
5. Serve each chaffle with tomato slices and basil leaves.

Nutrition:

Calories 67

Fat 5.6

Fiber 2

Carbs 4

Protein 2.1

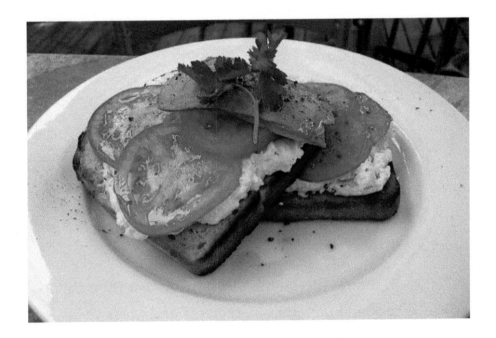

Spicy Black Sesame Chaffles

Preparation Time: 10 minutes

Cooking Time: 10 minutes

Servings: 4

Ingredients:

- 2 cups almond flour
- 2 cups almond milk
- Juice of 1/2 lemon
- 1/3 cup black sesame seeds
- A pinch of salt and black pepper
- 2 eggs, whisked
- 1 teaspoon chili powder
- 1 teaspoon hot paprika

Directions:

1. In a bowl merge the almond flour with the almond milk and the other ingredients and whisk well.
2. Heat up the Chaffle iron; pour 1/4 of the batter and cooking for 10 minutes.
3. Repeat with the rest of the mix and serve.

Nutrition:

Calories 69

Fat 4.9g

Fiber 2.1g

Carbs 5.4g

Protein 2.4g

Ham, Cheese & Tomato Chaffle Sandwich

Preparation time: 10 minutes

Cooking Time: 10 Minutes

Servings: 4

Ingredients:

- 1 teaspoon olive oil
- 2 slices ham
- 4 basic chaffles
- 1 tablespoon mayonnaise
- 2 slices Provolone cheese
- 1 tomato, sliced

Directions:

1. Attach the olive oil to a pan over medium heat.
2. Cook the ham for 1 minute per side.
3. Spread the chaffles with mayonnaise.
4. Top with the ham, cheese and tomatoes.
5. Top with another chaffle to make a sandwich.

Nutrition:

Calories: 13.3g

Saturated fat: 5.9g

Total carbs: 3.2g

Net carbs: 2.3g

Protein: 14.3g

Sugars: 1.4g

Salty Zucchini Onion Chaffles

Preparation Time: 5 minutes

Cooking Time: 7 minutes

Serving: 2

Ingredients:

- Egg: 1
- Mozzarella Cheese: 1/2 cup (shredded)
- Zucchini: 1/2 cup finely grated
- Onion: 1/2 cup chopped
- Garlic powder: 1/2 tsp.
- Pepper: 1/4 tsp.
- Salt: 1/4 tsp.

Direction:

1. Preheat a mini Chaffle maker if needed and grease it
2. Mix all the ingredients of the chaffle and mix well
3. Pour the mixture to the Chaffle maker
4. Cooking for at least 4 minutes to get the desired crunch and make as many chaffles as your batter allows

Nutrition

Calories: 341

Fat: 25g

Protein: 16g

Spiced Mozzarella Radish Chaffles

Preparation Time: 5 minutes

Cooking Time: 7 minutes

Serving: 2

Ingredients:

- Egg: 1
- Mozzarella cheese: 1/2 cup (shredded)
- Thyme: 1 tsp.
- Radish: 1/2 cup finely grated
- Allspice: a pinch
- Salt and pepper: as per your taste
- Coriander: 1/2 cup chopped

Direction:

1. Mix all the ingredients well together
2. Pour a layer on a preheated Chaffle iron
3. Cooking the chaffle for around 5 minutes
4. Make as many Chaffles as your mixture and Chaffle maker allow

Nutrition

Calories: 382

Fat: 31g

Protein: 21g

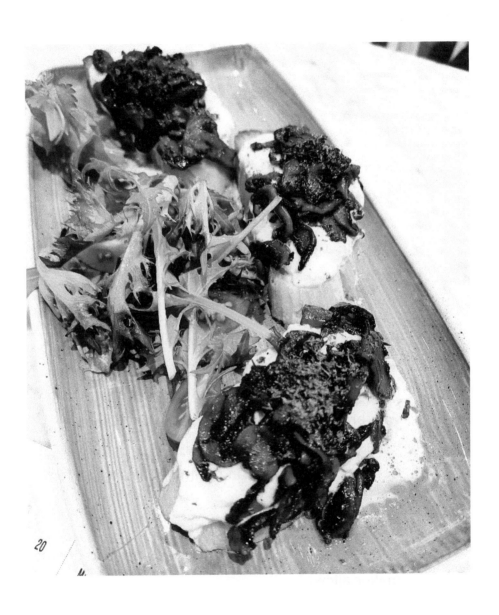

41

Boiled Broccoli Mozzarella Chaffles

Preparation Time: 25 minutes

Cooking Time: 7 minutes

Serving: 2

Ingredients:

- Eggs: 2
- Mozzarella: 1 cup shredded
- Cream cheese: 2 tbsp.
- Broccoli: 1 cup
- Salt: 1/4 tsp.

Direction:

1. Boil broccoli for 15 minutes in salted water
2. Preheat your mini Chaffle iron if needed
3. Mix all the above-mentioned ingredients in a bowl with broccoli and blend using a hand blender
4. Grease your Chaffle iron lightly
5. Cooking your mixture in the mini Chaffle iron for at least 4 minutes
6. Serve hot with your favorite sauce
7. Make as many Chaffles as your mixture and Chaffle maker allow

Nutrition

Calories: 370

Fat: 24g

Protein: 17g

Spinach Zucchini Chaffle

Preparation Time: 5 minutes

Cooking Time: 7 minutes

Serving: 2

Ingredients:

- Zucchini: 1 (small)
- Egg: 1
- Shredded mozzarella: half cup
- Parmesan: 1 tbsp.
- Pepper: As per your taste
- Basil: 1 tsp.
- Spinach: 1/2 cup

Direction:

1. Preheat your Chaffle iron
2. Grate zucchini finely
3. Boil spinach for five minutes and strain water
4. Add all the ingredients to zucchini in a bowl and mix well
5. Now add the spinach
6. Grease your Chaffle iron lightly
7. Pour the mixture into a full-size Chaffle maker and spread evenly
8. Cooking till it turns crispy

9. Make as many Chaffles as your mixture and Chaffle maker allow
10. Serve crispy and with your favorite keto sauce

Nutrition

Calories: 391

Fat: 31g

Protein: 29g

Crispy Carrot and Cabbage Chaffles

Preparation Time: 15 minutes

Cooking Time: 7 minutes

Serving: 2

Ingredients:

- Eggs: 2
- Mozzarella: 1 cup shredded
- Cream cheese: 2 tbsp.
- Butter: 1 tbsp.
- Onion: 1/2 cup
- Tomato: 1/2 cup
- Garlic powder: 1 tbsp.
- Pepper: 1/4 tsp.
- Basil: 1/2 tsp.
- Cabbage: 1/2 cup finely shredded
- Carrot: 1 cup sliced
- Salt: 1/4 tsp.

Direction:

1. Take a pan, heat butter and add onion and sauté for a minute
2. Add tomatoes and carrot and Cooking for 10 minutes
3. Preheat your mini Chaffle iron if needed

4. Mix all the above-mentioned ingredients in a bowl with carrots except for cabbage and blend using a hand blender
5. Add cabbage to the mixture from the top and mix
6. Grease your Chaffle iron lightly
7. Cooking your mixture in the mini Chaffle iron for at least 4 minutes
8. Serve hot with your favorite sauce
9. Make as many Chaffles as your mixture and Chaffle maker allow

Nutrition

Calories: 388

Fat: 29g

Protein: 11g

Okra Cauli Chaffle

Preparation Time: 5 minutes

Cooking Time: 7 minutes

Serving: 2

Ingredients:

- Cauliflower: 1/2 cup
- Okra: 1/2 cup
- Egg: 2
- Mozzarella Cheese: 1 cup (shredded)
- Butter: 1 tbsp.
- Almond flour: 2 tbsp.
- Turmeric: 1/4 tsp.
- Baking powder: 1/4 tsp.
- Onion powder: a pinch
- Garlic powder: a pinch
- Salt: a pinch

Direction:

1. In a deep saucepan, boil okra and cauliflower for five minutes or till it tenders, strain and set aside
2. Incorporate all the remaining ingredients well together
3. Fill in a thin layer on a preheated Chaffle iron
4. Take out any excess water from the vegetables and add a layer on the mixture

5. Again, add more mixture over the top

6. Cooking the chaffle for around 5 minutes

7. Serve hot with your favorite keto sauce

Nutrition

Calories: 332

Fat: 28.1g

Protein: 19.7g

Oniony Pickled Chaffles

Preparation Time: 25 minutes

Cooking Time: 7 minutes

Serving: 2

Ingredients:

- Egg: 1
- Onion: 1/2 cup finely chopped
- Cheddar Cheese: 1/2 cup (shredded)
- Pork panko: 1/2 cup
- Pickle slices: 6-8 thin
- Pickle juice: 1 tbsp.

Direction:

1. Mix egg, onion, cheese, and pork panko
2. Fill in a thin layer on a preheated Chaffle iron
3. Remove any excess juice from pickles
4. Add pickle slices and pour again more mixture over the top
5. Cooking the chaffle for around 5 minutes
6. Make as many Chaffles as your mixture and Chaffle maker allow

Nutrition

Calories: 366

Fat: 27g

Protein: 10g

Flavored Spinach Chaffles

Preparation Time: 5 minutes

Cooking Time: 7 minutes

Serving: 2

Ingredients:

- Egg: 1
- Cheddar Cheese: 1/2 cup (shredded)
- Thyme: 1 tsp.
- Spinach: 1/2 cup chopped
- Allspice: a pinch
- Salt and pepper: as per your taste
- Coriander: 1/2 cup chopped

Direction:

1. Mix all the ingredients well together
2. Pour a layer on a preheated Chaffle iron
3. Cooking the chaffle for around 5 minutes
4. Make as many Chaffles as your mixture and Chaffle maker allow

Nutrition

Calories: 391

Fat: 26g

Protein: 19.7g

Veggies and Olives Chaffles Salad

Preparation Time: 12 minutes

Cooking Time: 7 minutes

Serving: 2

Ingredients:

- Egg: 2
- Cheddar cheese: 1 cup (shredded)
- Onion: 1/2 cup thickly sliced
- Zucchini: 1/2 cup thickly sliced
- Cauliflower: 1 cup florets removed
- Salt: 1/2 tsp.
- Black pepper: 1/4 tsp.
- Butter: 1 tsp.
- Olives: 1/2 cup sliced
- Fresh coriander: 1/2 cup chopped

Direction:

1. Preheat the oven
2. Add all the vegetables on the baking tray and sprinkle salt and pepper
3. Brush with oil and roast for 15 min
4. Preheat a mini Chaffle maker if needed and grease it
5. Scourge eggs and sprinkle shredded cheddar cheese to them

6. Mix all well and fill the mixture to the lower plate of the Chaffle maker

7. Cooking for at least 4 minutes to get the desired crunch

8. Remove from the heat and divide into four pieces when cool down

9. Mix all the vegetable, olives, coriander, and chaffles together and serve

Nutrition

Calories: 391

Fat: 21g

Protein: 14g

Cauli Spinach Onion Blend Chaffles

Preparation Time: 25 minutes

Cooking Time: 7 minutes

Serving: 4

Ingredients:

- Eggs: 2
- Mozzarella: 1 cup shredded
- Cream cheese: 2 tbsp.
- Butter: 1 tbsp.
- Onion: 1/2 cup
- Tomato: 1/2 cup
- Garlic powder: 1 tbsp.
- Pepper: 1/4 tsp.
- Basil: 1/2 tsp.
- Spinach: 1/2 cup
- Cauliflower florets: 1 cup
- Salt: 1/4 tsp.

Direction:

1. Take a pan, heat butter and add onion and sauté for a minute
2. Add tomatoes, spinach, and cauliflower and Cooking for 10 minutes
3. Preheat your mini Chaffle iron if needed

4. Mix all the above-mentioned ingredients in a bowl with cauliflower and blend using a hand blender
5. Grease your Chaffle iron lightly
6. Cooking your mixture in the mini Chaffle iron for at least 4 minutes
7. Serve hot with your favorite sauce
8. Make as many Chaffles as your mixture and Chaffle maker allow

Nutrition

Calories: 377

Fat: 22g

Protein: 11g

Plain Spinach Jalapeno Chaffle

Preparation Time: 5 minutes

Cooking Time: 10 minutes

Serving: 2

Ingredients:

- Egg: 2
- Cheddar cheese: 11/2 cup
- Deli Jalapeno: 16 slices
- Spinach: 1 cup chopped

Direction:

1. Boil water and add spinach and boil for 5 minutes
2. Strain and drain to remove excess water
3. Preheat a mini Chaffle maker if needed
4. Scourge eggs and add half cheddar cheese to them and mix well
5. Shred some of the remaining cheddar cheese to the lower plate of the Chaffle maker
6. Now pour the mixture to the shredded cheese and add in one spoon of spinach and spread
7. Add the cheese again on the top with around 4 slices of jalapeno and close the lid
8. Cooking for at least 4 minutes to get the desired crunch and serve hot
9. Make as many Chaffles as your mixture allows

Nutrition

Calories: 339

Fat: 28.2g

Protein: 19g

Quick Onion Peppery Chaffles

Preparation Time: 5 minutes

Cooking Time: 7 minutes

Serving: 2

Ingredients:

- Egg: 1
- Mozzarella cheese: 1/2 cup (shredded)
- Garlic cloves: 2 chopped
- Pepper: 1/2 cup finely chopped
- Onion: 1/2 cup finely chopped
- Salt and pepper: as per your taste

Direction:

1. Mix all the ingredients well together
2. Pour a layer on a preheated Chaffle iron
3. Cooking the chaffle for around 5 minutes
4. Make as many Chaffles as your mixture and Chaffle maker allow

Nutrition

Calories: 347

Fat: 25g

Protein: 14g

Cauliflower & Italian Seasoning Chaffles

Preparation Time: 5 minutes

Cooking Time: 20 minutes

Serving: 4

Ingredients:

- 1 cup cauliflower rice
- 1/4 teaspoon garlic powder
- 1/2 teaspoon Italian seasoning
- Salt and freshly ground black pepper
- 1/2 cup Mexican blend cheese, shredded
- 1 organic egg, beaten
- 1/2 cup Parmesan cheese, shredded

Directions:

1. Preheat a mini Chaffle iron and then grease it.
2. In a blender, add all the ingredients except Parmesan cheese and pulse until well combined.
3. Place 11/2 tablespoon of the Parmesan cheese in the bottom of preheated Chaffle iron.
4. Place 1/4 of the egg mixture over cheese and sprinkle with the 1/2 tablespoon of the Parmesan cheese.
5. Cook for about 4-minutes or until golden brown.

6. Repeat with the remaining mixture and Parmesan cheese.

7. Serve warm.

Nutrition:

Calories: 127

Net Carb: 2gFat: 9g

Saturated Fat: 5.3g

Carbohydrates: 2.7g

Dietary Fiber: 0.7g

Sugar: 1.5g

Protein: 9.2g

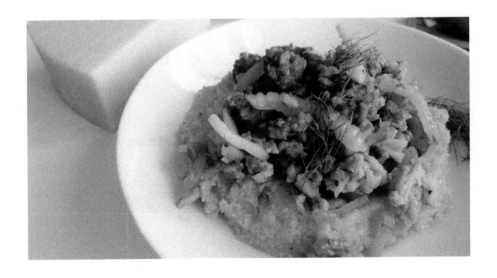

Pepperoni & Cauliflower Chaffles

Preparation Time: 5 minutes

Cooking Time: 16 minutes

Serving: 4

Ingredients:

- 6 turkey pepperoni slices, chopped
- 1/4 cup cauliflower rice
- 1 organic egg, beaten
- 1/4 cup Cheddar cheese, shredded
- 1/4 cup Mozzarella cheese, shredded
- 2 tablespoons Parmesan cheese, grated
- 1/2 teaspoon Italian seasoning
- 1/4 teaspoon onion powder
- 1/4 teaspoon garlic powder

Directions:

1. Preheat a mini Chaffle iron and then grease it.
2. In a medium bowl, set all ingredients and mix until well combined.
3. Place 1/4 of the mixture into preheated Chaffle iron and cook for about 4 minutes or until golden brown.
4. Repeat with the remaining mixture.
5. Serve warm.

Nutrition:

Calories: 103

Net Carb: 0.4g

Fat: 8gSaturated

Fat: 3.2g

Carbohydrates: 0.8g

Dietary Fiber: 0.2g

Sugar: 0.4g

Protein: 10.2g

Almond Spinach Chaffles

Preparation Time: 8 minutes

Cooking Time: 7 minutes

Serving: 2

Ingredients:

- Cheddar cheese: 1/3 cup
- Egg: 1
- Spinach: 1/3 cup finely chopped
- Lemon juice: 2 tbsp.
- Almond flour: 2 tbsp.
- Baking powder: 1/4 teaspoon
- Ground almonds: 2 tbsp.
- Mozzarella cheese: 1/3 cup

Direction:

1. Mix cheddar cheese, egg, lemon juice, spinach, almond flour, almond ground, and baking powder together in a bowl
2. Preheat your Chaffle iron and grease it
3. In your mini Chaffle iron, shred half of the mozzarella cheese
4. Add the mixture to your mini Chaffle iron
5. Again, shred the remaining mozzarella cheese on the mixture
6. Cooking till the desired crisp is achieved

7. Make as many chaffles as your mixture and Chaffle maker allow

Nutrition

Calories: 342

Fat: 24g

Protein: 19.7g

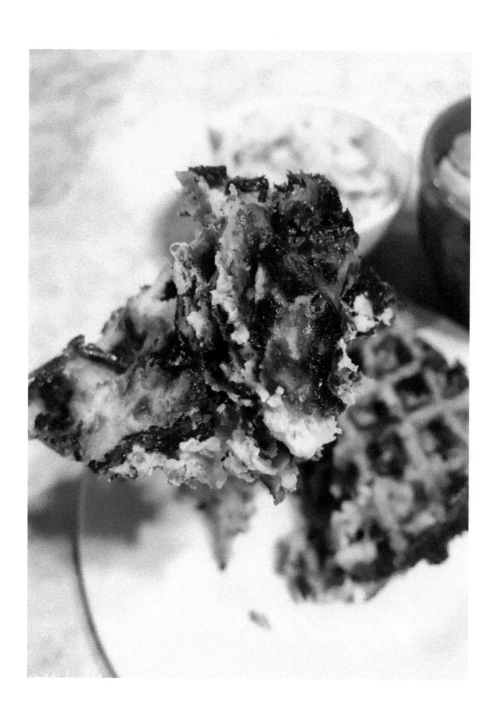

Okra Fritter Chaffle

Preparation Time: 15 minutes

Cooking Time: 7 minutes

Serving: 2

Ingredients:

- Egg: 1
- Mozzarella cheese: 1/4 cup
- Onion powder: 1/2 tbsp.
- Heavy cream: 2 tbsp.
- Mayo: 1 tbsp.
- Garlic: 2 cloves (finely chopped)
- Almond flour: 1/4 cup
- Okra: 1 cup
- Salt: 1/4 tsp. or as per your taste
- Black pepper: 1/4 tsp.

Direction:

1. Combine egg, mayo, and heavy cream and whisk
2. When mixed, add almond flour and make a uniform batter
3. Leave it for 5-10 minutes
4. Now add okra and rest of the ingredients and mix well
5. Preheat a mini Chaffle maker if needed and grease it

6. Pour the mixture to the lower plate of the Chaffle maker and spread it evenly to cover the plate properly
7. Cooking for at least 4 minutes to get the desired crunch
8. Remove the chaffle from the heat
9. Make as many chaffles as your mixture and Chaffle maker allow
10. Serve hot and enjoy!

Nutrition

Calories: 339

Fat: 28g

Protein: 19g

Carbs: 3 g

Spiced Spinach, Carrot, and Onion Chaffles

Preparation Time: 5 minutes

Cooking Time: 17 minutes

Serving: 2

Ingredients:

- Eggs: 2
- Mozzarella: 1 cup shredded
- Cream cheese: 2 tbsp.
- Butter: 1 tbsp.
- Onion: 1/2 cup
- Tomato: 1/2 cup
- Garlic powder: 1 tbsp.
- Pepper: 1/4 tsp.
- Basil: 1/2 tsp.
- Spinach: 1/2 cup chopped
- Carrot: 1 cup sliced
- Salt: 1/4 tsp.

Direction:

1. Take a pan, heat butter and add onion and sauté for a minute
2. Add tomatoes, spinach, and carrot and Cooking for 10 minutes

3. Preheat your mini Chaffle iron if needed
4. Mix all the above-mentioned ingredients in a bowl with carrots and blend using a hand blender
5. Grease your Chaffle iron lightly
6. Cooking your mixture in the mini Chaffle iron for at least 4 minutes
7. Serve hot with your favorite sauce
8. Make as many chaffles as your mixture and Chaffle maker allow

Nutrition

Calories: 339

Fat: 24g

Protein: 17g

Carbs: 1.3 g

Spiced Coriander Chaffle

Preparation Time: 5 minutes

Cooking Time: 7 minutes

Serving: 2

Ingredients:

- Egg: 1
- Cheddar Cheese: 1/2 cup (shredded)
- Thyme: 1 tsp.
- Allspice: a pinch
- Salt and pepper: as per your taste
- Coriander: 1/2 cup chopped

Direction:

1. Mix all the ingredients well together
2. Pour a layer on a preheated Chaffle iron
3. Cooking the chaffle for around 5 minutes
4. Make as many chaffles as your mixture and Chaffle maker allow

Nutrition

Calories: 329

Fat: 25g

Protein: 16g

Carbs: 1.9

Pickled Spinach Chaffles

Preparation Time: 15 minutes

Cooking Time: 7 minutes

Serving: 2

Ingredients:

- Egg: 1
- Spinach: 1/2 cup chopped, boiled, and drained
- Cheddar Cheese: 1/2 cup (shredded)
- Pork panko: 1/2 cup
- Pickle slices: 6-8 thin

Direction:

1. Mix egg, spinach, cheese, and pork panko
2. Fill in a thin layer on a preheated Chaffle iron
3. Remove any excess juice from pickles
4. Add pickle slices and pour again more mixture over the top
5. Cooking the chaffle for around 5 minutes
6. Make as many chaffles as your mixture and Chaffle maker allow

Nutrition

Calories: 394

Fat: 28g

Protein: 11g

Carbs: 3 g

Mushroom and Almond Chaffle

Preparation Time: 5 minutes

Cooking Time: 15 minutes

Serving: 4

Ingredients:

Batter

- 4 eggs
- 2 cups grated mozzarella cheese
- 1 cup finely chopped zucchini
- 3 tablespoons chopped almonds
- 2 teaspoons baking powder
- Salt and pepper to taste
- 1 teaspoon dried basil
- 1 teaspoon chili flakes

Other

- 2 tablespoons Cooking spray to brush the Chaffle maker

Directions

1. Preheat the Chaffle maker.

2. Add the eggs, grated mozzarella, mushrooms, almonds, baking powder, salt and pepper, dried basil and chili flakes to a bowl.
3. Mix with a fork.
4. Brush the heated Chaffle maker with Cooking spray and add a few tablespoons of the batter.
5. Close the lid and Cooking for about 5–7 minutes depending on your Chaffle maker.
6. Serve and enjoy.

Nutrition

Calories 196

Fat 16 G

Carbs 4 G

Sugar 1 G,

Protein 10.8 G

Sodium 152 Mg

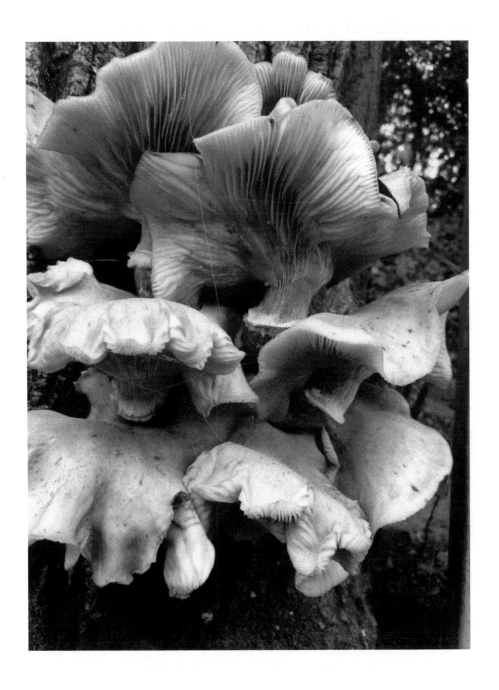

Avocado Croquet Madam Chaffle

Preparation Time: 5 minutes

Cooking Time: 15 minutes

Serving: 4

Ingredients:

Batter

- 4 eggs
- 2 cups grated mozzarella cheese
- 1 avocado, mashed
- Salt and pepper to taste
- 6 tablespoons almond flour
- 2 teaspoons baking powder
- 1 teaspoon dried dill

Other

- 2 tablespoons Cooking spray to brush the Chaffle maker
- 4 fried eggs
- 2 tablespoons freshly chopped basil

Directions

1. Preheat the Chaffle maker.
2. Add the eggs, grated mozzarella, avocado, salt and pepper, almond flour, baking powder and dried dill to a bowl.

3. Mix with a fork.
4. Brush the heated Chaffle maker with Cooking spray and add a few tablespoons of the batter.
5. Close the lid and Cooking for about 5–7 minutes depending on your Chaffle maker.
6. Serve each chaffle with a fried egg and freshly chopped basil on top.

Nutrition

Calories 393

Fat 32.1 G

Carbs 9.2 G

Sugar 1.3 G,

Protein 18.8 G

Sodium 245 Mg

Spinach and Artichoke Chaffle

Preparation Time: 5 minutes

Cooking Time: 15 minutes

Serving: 4

Ingredients:

Batter

- 4 eggs
- 2 cups grated provolone cheese
- 1 cup Cooked and diced spinach
- 1/2 cup diced artichoke hearts
- Salt and pepper to taste
- 2 tablespoons coconut flour
- 2 teaspoons baking powder

Other

- 2 tablespoons Cooking spray to brush the Chaffle maker
- 1/4 cup of cream cheese for serving

Directions

1. Preheat the Chaffle maker.
2. Add the eggs, grated provolone cheese, diced spinach, artichoke hearts, salt and pepper, coconut flour and baking powder to a bowl.
3. Mix with a fork.

4. Brush the heated Chaffle maker with Cooking spray and add a few tablespoons of the batter.
5. Close the lid and Cooking for about 5–7 minutes depending on your Chaffle maker.
6. Serve each chaffle with cream cheese.

Nutrition

Calories 427

Fat 32.8 g

Carbs 9.5 g,

Sugar 1.1 g

Protein 25.7 g

Sodium 722 Mg

Asparagus Chaffle

Preparation Time: 5 minutes

Cooking Time: 15 minutes

Serving: 4

Ingredients:

Batter

- 4 eggs
- 11/2 cups grated mozzarella cheese
- 1/2 cup grated parmesan cheese
- 1 cup boiled asparagus, chopped
- Salt and pepper to taste
- 1/4 cup almond flour
- 2 teaspoons baking powder

Other

- 2 tablespoons Cooking spray to brush the Chaffle maker
- 1/4 cup Greek yogurt for serving
- 1/4 cup chopped almonds for serving

Directions

1. Preheat the Chaffle maker.
2. Add the eggs, grated mozzarella, grated parmesan, asparagus, salt and pepper, almond flour and baking powder to a bowl.

3. Mix with a fork.
4. Brush the heated Chaffle maker with Cooking spray and add a few tablespoons of the batter.
5. Close the lid and Cooking for about 5–7 minutes depending on your Chaffle maker.
6. Serve each chaffle with Greek yogurt and chopped almonds.

Nutrition

Calories 316

Fat 24.9 g

Carbs 7.3 g,

Sugar 1.2 g,

Protein 18.2 g

Sodium 261 Mg

Broccoli Chaffle

Preparation Time: 5 minutes

Cooking Time: 15 minutes

Serving: 4

Ingredients:

Batter

- 4 eggs
- 2 cups grated mozzarella cheese
- 1 cup steamed broccoli, chopped
- Salt and pepper to taste
- 1 clove garlic, minced
- 1 teaspoon chili flakes
- 2 tablespoons almond flour
- 2 teaspoons baking powder

Other

- 2 tablespoons Cooking spray to brush the Chaffle maker
- 1/4 cup mascarpone cheese for serving

Directions

1. Preheat the Chaffle maker.
2. Add the eggs, grated mozzarella, chopped broccoli, salt and pepper, minced garlic, chili flakes, almond flour and baking powder to a bowl.

82

3. Mix with a fork.
4. Brush the heated Chaffle maker with Cooking spray and add a few tablespoons of the batter.
5. Close the lid and Cooking for about 5–7 minutes depending on your Chaffle maker.
6. Serve each chaffle with mascarpone cheese.

Nutrition

Calories 229

Fat 17.5 g

Carbs 6 g

Sugar 1.1 g

Protein 13.1 g

Sodium 194 Mg

Cauliflower Chaffle

Preparation Time: 5 minutes

Cooking Time: 15 minutes

Serving: 4

Ingredients:

Batter

- 4 eggs
- 2 cups grated cheddar cheese
- 1 cup steamed cauliflower, chopped
- Salt and pepper to taste
- 1 teaspoon dried basil
- 1/2 teaspoon onion powder
- 2 tablespoons almond flour
- 2 teaspoons baking powder

Other

- 2 tablespoons Cooking spray to brush the Chaffle maker
- 1/4 cup mascarpone cheese for serving

Directions

1. Preheat the Chaffle maker.
2. Add the eggs, grated cheddar, cauliflower, salt and pepper, dried basil, onion powder, almond flour and baking powder to a bowl.

3. Mix with a fork.
4. Brush the heated Chaffle maker with Cooking spray and add a few tablespoons of the batter.
5. Close the lid and Cooking for about 5–7 minutes depending on your Chaffle maker.
6. Serve each chaffle with mascarpone cheese.

Nutrition

Calories 409

Fat 33.7 g,

Carbs 5 g

Sugar 1.4 g,

Protein 22.7 g

Sodium 434 Mg

Celery and Cottage Cheese Chaffle

Preparation Time: 5 minutes

Cooking Time: 15 minutes

Serving: 4

Ingredients:

Batter

- 4 eggs
- 2 cups grated cheddar cheese
- 1 cup fresh celery, chopped
- Salt and pepper to taste
- 2 tablespoons chopped almonds
- 2 teaspoons baking powder

Other

- 2 tablespoons Cooking spray to brush the Chaffle maker
- 1/4 cup cottage cheese for serving

Directions

1. Preheat the Chaffle maker.
2. Add the eggs, grated mozzarella cheese, chopped celery, salt and pepper, chopped almonds and baking powder to a bowl.
3. Mix with a fork.

4. Brush the heated Chaffle maker with Cooking spray and add a few tablespoons of the batter.
5. Close the lid and Cooking for about 5–7 minutes depending on your Chaffle maker.
6. Serve each chaffle with cottage cheese on top.

Nutrition

Calories 385

Fat 31.6 G

Carbs 4 G

Sugar 1.5 G,

Protein 22.2 G

Sodium 492 Mg

Garlic and Spinach Chaffles

Preparation Time 5 minutes

Cooking time 5minutes

Servings 2

Ingredients

- 1 cup egg whites
- 1 tsp. Italian spice
- 2 tsps. coconut flour
- 1/2 tsp. vanilla
- 1 tsp. baking powder
- 1 tsp. baking soda
- 1 cup mozzarella cheese, grated
- 1/2 tsp. garlic powder
- 1 cup chopped spinach

Directions

1. Switch on your square Chaffle maker. Spray with non-stick spray.
2. Beat egg whites with beater, until fluffy and white.
3. Add pumpkin puree, pumpkin pie spice, and coconut flour in egg whites and beat again.
4. Stir in the cheese, powder, garlic powder, baking soda, and powder.
5. Sprinkle chopped spinach on a Chaffle maker

6. Pour the batter in Chaffle maker over chopped spinach
7. Close the maker and Cooking for about 4-5 minutes.
8. Remove chaffles from the maker.
9. Serve hot and enjoy!

Nutrition

Total Calories 173 kcal

Fats 7.71 g

Protein 21.31 g

Net Carbs 2.02g

Fiber 0.3 g

Starch 0 g

Vegan Chaffles With Flaxseed

Preparation Time: 5 minutes

Cooking time: 5minutes

Servings 2

Ingredients

- 1 tbsp. flaxseed meal
- 2 tbsps. warm water
- 1/4 cup low carb vegan cheese
- 1/4 cup chopped mint
- pinch of salt
- 2 oz. blueberries chunks

Directions

1. Preheat Chaffle maker to medium-high heat and grease with Cooking spray.
2. Mix together flaxseed meal and warm water and set aside to be thickened.
3. After 5 minutes' mix together all ingredients in flax egg.
4. Pour vegan Chaffle batter into the center of the Chaffle iron.
5. Close the Chaffle maker and let Cooking for 3-5 minutes
6. Once Cooked, remove the vegan chaffle from the Chaffle maker and serve.

Nutrition

Total Calories 130 kcal

Fats 42.44 g

Protein 10.1 g

Net Carbs 1.6 g

Fiber 1.4 g

Almonds and Flaxseeds Chaffles

Preparation Time 5 minutes

Cooking time 5minutes

Servings 2

Ingredients

- 1/4 cup coconut flour
- 1 tsp. stevia
- 1 tbsp. ground flaxseed
- 1/4 tsp. baking powder
- 1/2 cup almond milk
- 1/4 tsp. vanilla extract
- 1/2 cup low carb vegan cheese

Directions

1. Mix together flaxseed in warm water and set aside.
2. Add in the remaining ingredients.
3. Switch on Chaffle iron and grease with cooking spray.
4. Pour the batter in the Chaffle machine and close the lid.
5. Cooking the chaffles for about 3-4 minutes.
6. Once cooked, remove from the Chaffle machine.
7. Serve with berries and enjoy!

Nutrition

Total Calories 130 kcal

Fats 42.44 g

Protein 10.1 g

Net Carbs 1.6 g

Fiber 1.4 g

Starch 0 g

Vegan Chocolate Chaffles

Preparation Time 5 minutes

Cooking time 5minutes

Servings 2

Ingredients

- 1/2 cup coconut flour
- 3 tbsps. cocoa powder
- 2 tbsps. whole psyllium husk
- 1/2 teaspoon baking powder
- pinch of salt
- 1/2 cup vegan cheese, softened
- 1/4 cup coconut milk

Directions

1. Set your Chaffle iron according to the manufacturer's Directions.
2. Mix together coconut flour, cocoa powder, baking powder, salt and husk in a bowl and set aside.
3. Add melted cheese and milk and mix well. Let it stand for a few minutes before Cooking.
4. Pour batter in Chaffle machine and Cooking for about 3-4 minutes.
5. Once chaffles are cooked, carefully remove them from the Chaffle machine.
6. Serve with vegan ice cream and enjoy!

Nutrition

Calories 130 kcal

Fats 42.44 g

Protein 10.1 g

Net Carbs 1.6 g

Fiber 1.4 g

Starch 0 g

Garlic Mayo Vegan Chaffles

Preparation Time 5 minutes

Cooking time 5minutes

Servings: 2

Ingredients

- 1 tbsp. chia seeds
- 2 1/2 tbsps. water
- 1/4 cup low carb vegan cheese
- 2 tbsps. coconut flour
- 1 cup low carb vegan cream cheese, softened
- 1 tsp. garlic powder
- pinch of salt
- 2 tbsps. vegan garlic mayo for topping

Directions

1. Preheat your square Chaffle maker.
2. In a small bowl, merge chia seeds and water; let it stand for 5 minutes.
3. Add all ingredients to the chia seeds mixture and mix well.
4. Pour vegan chaffle batter in a greased Chaffle maker
5. Close the Chaffle maker and Cooking for about 3-5 minutes.
6. Once chaffles are Cooked, remove from the maker.

7. Top with garlic mayo and pepper.

8. Enjoy!

Nutrition

Calories 130 kcal

Fats 42.44 g

Protein 10.1 g

Net Carbs 1.6 g

Fiber 1.4 g

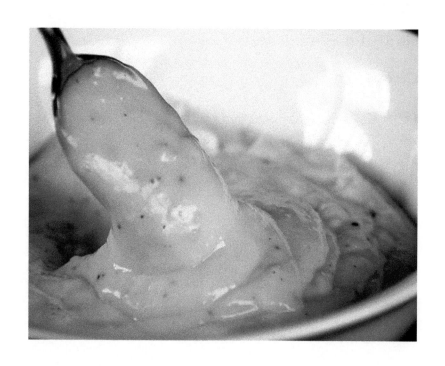

Crispy Cauli Chaffle

Preparation Time 5 minutes

Cooking time 10 minutes

Servings: 2

Ingredients

- Cauliflower rice: 1 cup
- Egg: 1
- Parmesan cheese: 1/2 cup (shredded)
- Mozzarella Cheese: 1/2 cup (shredded)
- Salt: 1/4 tsp. or as per your taste
- Black pepper: 1/4 tsp.
- Italian seasoning: 1/2 tsp.
- Garlic powder: 1/2 tsp.

Directions:

1. Preheat a mini Chaffle maker if needed and grease it
2. Add all the ingredients, except for parmesan cheese, into a blender
3. Mix them all well
4. Spread 1/8 cup of shredded parmesan cheese to the lower plate of the Chaffle maker
5. Pour the cauliflower mixture above the cheese
6. Again sprinkle 1/8 cup of shredded parmesan cheese on top of the mixture

7. Close the lid

8. Cook for at least 5 minutes to get the desired crunch

9. Remove the chaffle from the heat

10. Serve hot and enjoy!

Nutrition

Calories: 394

Fat: 28g

Protein: 11g

Carbs: 3 g

Jicama Loaded Chaffle

Preparation Time 5 minutes

Cooking time 10 minutes

Servings: 2

Ingredients

- Egg: 2
- Cheddar cheese: 1 cup
- Onion: 1/2 medium minced
- Jicama root: 1 large
- Garlic: 2 cloves
- Salt: 1/4 tsp. or as per your taste
- Black pepper: 1/4 tsp.

Directions:

1. With peeler or knife, peel jicama and blend it in a food processor
2. Put this in a large colander with a pinch of salt and let it drain
3. Make it dry as much as possible
4. Microwave it for around 7 minutes
5. Now add the remaining ingredients to the blended jicama and mix well
6. Preheat a mini Chaffle maker if needed and grease it

7. Pour the mixture to the lower plate of the Chaffle maker and spread it evenly to cover the plate properly
8. Close the lid
9. Cook for at least 4 minutes to get the desired crunch
10. Remove the chaffle from the heat
11. Make as many chaffles as your mixture and Chaffle maker allow
12. Serve hot and enjoy!

Nutrition:

Calories: 121kcal

Carbohydrates: 3g

Protein: 9g

Fat: 8g

Spinach Garlic Butter Chaffle

Preparation Time 15 minutes

Cooking time 20 minutes

Servings: 2

Ingredients

For the Chaffle:

- Egg: 2
- Mozzarella Cheese: 1 cup (shredded)
- Garlic powder: 1/2 tsp.
- Italian seasoning: 1 tsp.
- Cream cheese: 1 tsp.
- Spinach: 1/2 cup

For the Garlic Butter Topping:

- Garlic powder: 1/2 tsp.
- Italian seasoning: 1/2 tsp.
- Butter: 1 tbsp.

Directions:

1. In a small saucepan, attach 1/4 cup water with spinach and simmer for 5 minutes
2. Drain the excess water from spinach and set aside
3. Preheat a mini Chaffle maker if needed and grease it

4. In a mixing bowl, attach all the ingredients of the chaffle along with the prepared spinach and mix well

5. Pour the mixture to the lower plate of the Chaffle maker and spread it evenly to cover the plate properly and close the lid

6. Cook for at least 4 minutes to get the desired crunch

7. In the meanwhile, melt butter and add the garlic butter ingredients

8. Remove the chaffle from the heat and apply the garlic butter immediately

9. Make as many chaffles as your mixture and Chaffle maker allow

Nutrition

Calories 427

Fat 32.8 g

Carbs 9.5 g,

Sugar 1.1 g

Protein 25.7 g

Crispy Bagel Chaffles

Preparation time: 5 minutes

Cooking Time: 30 Minutes

Servings: 2

Ingredients:

- 2 eggs
- 1/2 cup parmesan cheese
- 1 tsp. bagel seasoning
- 1/2 cup mozzarella cheese
- 2 teaspoons almond flour

Directions:

1. Turn on Chaffle maker to heat and oil it with Cooking spray.
2. Evenly sprinkle half of cheeses to a griddle and let them melt. Then toast for 30 seconds and leave them wait for batter.
3. Whisk eggs, other half of cheeses, almond flour, and bagel seasoning in a small bowl.
4. Pour batter into the Chaffle maker. Cooking for minutes.
5. Let cool for 2-3 minutes before serving.

Nutrition:

Calories 117

Fat 2.1g

Carbs 18.2g,

Protein 22.7g

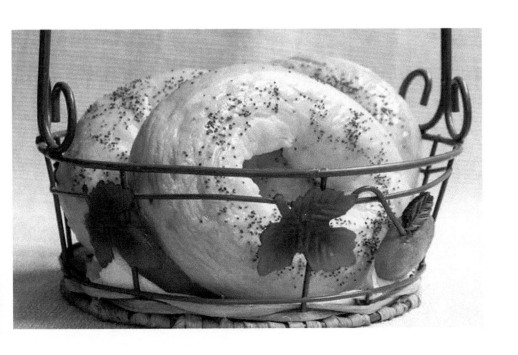